MAKE it WORK!
BODY

Andrew Haslam

written by
Liz Wyse

Photography: Jon Barnes
Science Consultant: Sue Dale Tunnicliffe
Primary Science & Technology Executive Officer
International Council of Associations for Science Education

Scholastic Canada Ltd.,
123 Newkirk Road, Richmond Hill, Ontario, Canada L4C 3G5

MAKE it WORK!

Other titles

Building
Earth
Electricity
Flight
Insects
Machines
Plants
Sound
Space

Published in Canada in 1995 by
Scholastic Canada Ltd.,
123 Newkirk Road, Richmond Hill, Ontario, Canada L4C 3G5

First published in Great Britain in 1994 by
Two-Can Publishing Ltd,
346 Old Street, London EC1V 9NQ

Copyright © Two-Can Publishing Ltd, 1994
Design of models © Andrew Haslam, 1994

Printed and bound in Hong Kong

2 4 6 8 10 9 7 5 3 1

All rights reserved. No part of this publication may be reproduced, stored in a retrieval system or transmitted in any form or by any means electronic, mechanical, photocopying, recording or otherwise, without prior written permission of the copyright owner.

Canadian Cataloguing in Publication Data

Haslam, Andrew
   Body

(Make it work!)
Includes index.
ISBN 0-590-24333-0 (bound)   ISBN 0-590-24614-3 (pbk.)

1. Body, Human – Juvenile literature. 2. Human physiology – Juvenile literature. I. Wyse Liz. II. Title. III. Series.

QP37.H37   1994   j612   C94-930774-2

Editor: Lucy Duke
Series concept and design: Andrew Haslam and Wendy Baker
Assistant model-maker: Sarah Davies
Additional design: Lisa Nutt and Helen McDonagh

Thanks also to:
Colin and Jenny at Plough Studios, Rachel, Katharine and Jonathan Bee, Tony Ellis, Richard Scarlett, Alison and Elizabeth Bricknell, Wen-Hshin Chen and Ajitha Ranasinghe.

Contents

Being a Scientist	4
The Skeleton	6
The Skull	8
Joints	10
Muscles	12
Skin	14
Cells	16
The Nervous System	18
Blood	20
The Heart	22
The Lungs	24
Digestion	26
Purification	30
The Brain	32
Memory	34
Sight	36
Taste and Smell	38
Touch and Hearing	40
Reproduction	42
The Whole Body	44
Glossary	46
Index	48

Words marked in **bold** in the text are explained in the glossary.

4 Being a Scientist

Did you know that your body contains over 200 bones and over 600 muscles, or that your heart beats 100,000 times a day and never rests? Do you realize that your body is about 70 per cent water? The human body is a fascinating world just waiting to be explored.

What are humans?

Human beings belong to the big group of animals called mammals. We share a number of important characteristics with other mammals. We have a bony skeleton, which is inside our body. We are warm-blooded, which means that our body controls its own temperature. And we give birth to live young and feed our babies on milk made inside the mother's body.

*All human beings belong to a **species**, or group, called* Homo sapiens, *or 'wise man'.*

Biologists are scientists who examine the living world. All living things, including human beings, share certain characteristics. They take in food and use the chemical energy they obtain from it to help them grow and move. They make waste products. They respond to the world around them. They all start out as a single **cell**, and reproduce to create new life.

A crafty tip

To paint your body models, use acrylic paint or mix ordinary paint with rubber solution glue.

MAKE it WORK!

Become a human biologist. Take a closer look at yourself and the people around you. You can try the experiments in this book on yourself or your friends. Many of the activities will show you the world that lies beneath your skin, so you can find out what happens under the surface. There are also models to make that help you understand how important **organs**, such as your heart and lungs, actually work.

Modelling the body

You will be making life-size models of all the body's main systems. Eventually, you will see your own body 'inside out'! The pictures show you some of the equipment you will need.

Doing experiments

Several experiments will show you how your body works. As a scientist, you must be careful to keep a record of all your experiments. You can do this by writing notes, or you could record your findings on a tape recorder. The main equipment and tools you will need for your experiments is shown in the picture.

Did you know you are the end result of up to 1 1/2 million years of human history? In this time, humans have changed and developed. We have learned to walk upright and use our hands to work with tools. We also use language to communicate with each other.

6 The Skeleton

Your **skeleton** is your body's framework. It is made up of 206 bones, which meet and link up at **joints**. Your bones come in many different sizes and shapes, depending on the jobs they have to do. The largest bone in the human body is the thigh bone or femur. The smallest is a tiny bone inside the ear called the stirrup.

Standing up straight
Most mammals move along on all fours. Our human skeleton, helped by our **muscles** and **ligaments**, allows us to walk around while we are still standing up straight. The long, thick bones of our legs and feet carry the weight of our bodies. The bowl-shaped bones of the pelvis (or hips) are a firm base for the spine (or backbone).

MAKE it WORK!
Have you ever wondered what it would be like to see through your skin and muscles to the skeleton underneath? Make your own bones from cut-out cardboard, stick them in position and turn yourself into a real live skeleton!

You will need
a pair of scissors
double-sided sticky tape
paints or coloured pencils
sheets of light-coloured cardboard

▲ Humans have short, stiff toes which act as a strong springy base, pushing the body off the ground as we walk along and helping balance.

1 Following the photographs above, draw all the bone shapes on the cardboard. Try to measure them to fit your body.

2 Cut out the bone shapes.

3 Use paints or pencils to colour the bones – make them darker around the joints (where two bones meet).

The protecting skeleton
Some bones protect the organs inside our bodies. The rounded shape of the pelvis guards the bladder. Ribs surround the heart and lungs like the curved bars of a cage, and the skull protects the brain.

All mammals have more or less the same number of bones in their bodies, whatever their size. A mouse has just as many bones as an elephant.

▲ Humans have extra-long, flexible thumbs, which can touch each fingertip in turn. Long thumbs mean that our hands can grip large objects, as well as carrying out more delicate jobs such as threading needles.

4 Put on some old, plain-coloured clothes. Then ask a friend to help you stick the skeleton to your body using double-sided sticky tape.

5 When you come to the bones of the upper body, stick the spine and shoulder blades on first. The ribs fit in a curve around the spine.

Living bones
Did you know that bones are actually alive? If they are cracked or broken they can mend themselves. They simply make new bone tissue which knits together the gap made by the break.

The hard outer case of a bone surrounds a spongy inside. Some bones also contain a jelly-like substance called **marrow**. *Bone marrow is vitally important for a healthy body because it makes new red blood cells.*

8 The Skull

Your skull is a hard case made of bone which protects your brain and your sense organs. Eight strong, bony plates at the top of your skull are joined together, curving around your brain. The bones of your lower skull protect your eyes and ears. Your teeth are fixed firmly in small holes in your upper and lower jawbones.

A crafty tip For some activities in this book, you will need to cut out quite difficult cardboard shapes. If anyone has a photocopier you can use, you could copy the shapes onto tracing paper, enlarge them on the photocopier, then cut out the photocopies to make full-size templates.

1 Cut out the skull shape from the cardboard.

2 Copy the wavy lines shown in the photograph. These lines on the skull are called sutures. They show where the bones have fused together.

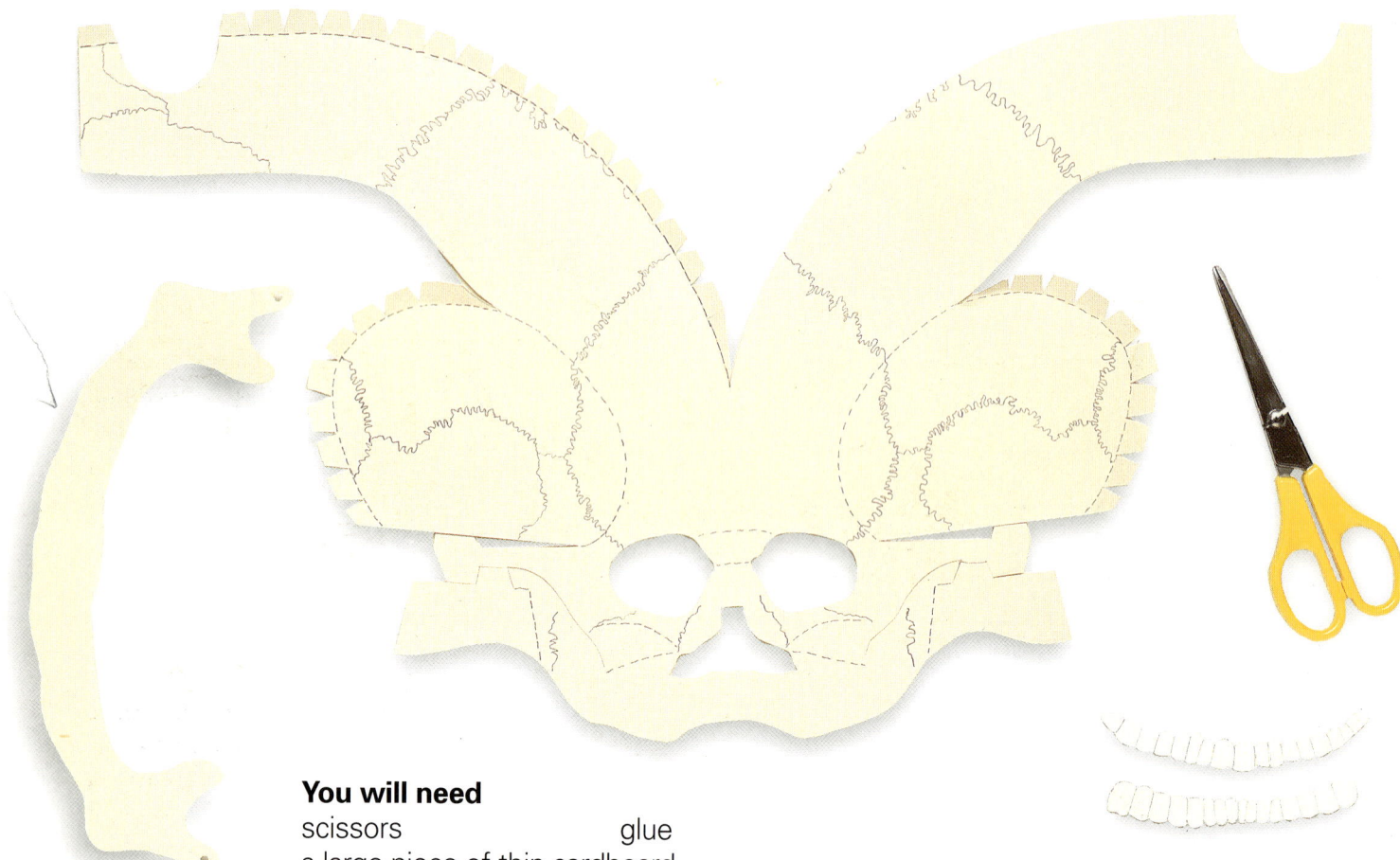

You will need
scissors   glue
a large piece of thin cardboard
two paper fasteners

MAKE it WORK!
Make your own cardboard skull, complete with hinged jawbone, and see for yourself exactly how the fixed bones of the upper skull fit together. You will notice that the jawbone is the only part of the skull which can actually move.

When you were born, your skull was soft because the bones were still forming. By the time you were two, the separate bones had hardened and knitted together. The lines where they joined are visible on the skull. As you get older, these lines begin to fade and may disappear altogether.

5 Join the jawbone to either side of the skull, using the two paper fasteners.

6 Finally, glue all thirty-two teeth in place, one set on the upper jaw and one on the lower jaw. You should now have a grinning skull!

3 Cut along the solid lines to make tabs. Score and fold along the dotted lines.

4 Glue the tabs along the top and sides of the skull.

eyeballs protected by the eye sockets

ear canal leads inwards to the inner ear

teeth

hinged joint attaches the jawbone to the skull

jawbone

There are 22 bones in your skull altogether and 14 of these are in your face. Your nose and your ears are not made of bone and so they are not part of your skull. Softer, flexible **tissue** *called cartilage gives them their shape.*

10 Joints

Where two bones meet, they form a joint. Our joints let us bend, twist and turn our bodies. At the joint, the bones are cushioned from each other by soft, protective tissue called cartilage, and also by a special fluid which prevents them from grinding against each other. Ligaments act like stretchy straps to hold the bones together.

You will need

polystyrene blocks felt-tip pens
acrylic paint a craft file

1 Draw the shapes of the joints on the polystyrene as shown. Use a craft file to carve them out, using the lines as guides.

2 Paint the finished joints creamy yellow.

Fused joints The joints of your skull are fused together, like the pieces of a jigsaw. They form a solid bony plate which protects your brain.

axis

atlas

skull

MAKE it WORK!
You have many types of joints in your body. Each is specially designed for different kinds of movement. Joints help you to hold your head upright, walk, and use your hands and fingers in many different ways. Make these models and find out how the joint matches the movement.

Cartilaginous joints Your spine has 24 bones. The joints between them are called cartilaginous joints. They allow your spine to be flexible.

◀ **Pivot joints** In your neck you have a pivot joint, which lets you nod and shake your head. The atlas bone rotates around the axis bone at the top of your spine to make this special joint.

Look at your own body, and see how your joints work. It is easy to see, for example, that your elbow has a hinge joint. Compare the range of movement in your elbow with your shoulder, which has a different, more flexible joint.

An average person flexes their finger joints 25 million times in their life! Not surprisingly, the joints can wear out. They become swollen and painful. This is called osteo-arthritis.

ball and socket joint

hinge joint

thumb joint

Ball and socket joint The end of one bone is ball-shaped and swivels around in the cup-shaped socket bone. Ball and socket joints are found in your hips and shoulders. Very supple people have a great range of movement in these joints.

Hinge joint These are joints which move back and forth in a straight line, like the hinges on a door. You will find this kind of joint in your elbows and knees.

Thumb joint The lowest bone in your thumb (the **metacarpal**) has a little lip at the end. This slots neatly into the small bone at the base of your thumb. When these two bones work together they give your thumb completely circular movement.

12 Muscles

The bones of the skeleton are moved by muscles. The human body has about 600 **skeletal** muscles. These move because you decide they should. Other **involuntary** muscles, such as those in your digestive system, move when your body needs them to work.

You will need

a hinge
a screwdriver
three strips of wood
two red and two green elastic bands
four screws
seven open hooks
two closed hooks

MAKE it WORK!

Muscles are joined to bones by **tendons**, which are like strips of elastic. They work by pulling against the bone to which they are attached. Make your own working muscle model, and see for yourself how strong your muscles have to be.

1 Use the screwdriver to screw the hinge onto one end of the wider piece of wood. Screw the two narrower pieces to the other half of the hinge. The pieces of wood represent the three bones of your arm. You can compare them with the arm bones you made on page 6.

2 Twist four of the open hooks and one closed hook into the wood as shown. Thread the red elastic bands through the closed hook and stretch them between the open hooks. These bands represent the biceps, which is the muscle inside your upper arm.

3 Screw in the remaining hooks as shown and attach green elastic bands to form the triceps, the muscle on the outside of your upper arm.

Your completed working model shows you how muscles often work in pairs (represented by the different-coloured bands). One muscle contracts, or gets shorter and fatter. As it shortens, it pulls the bone it is attached to, bending the joint. The other muscle in the pair works in the same way to straighten the joint out. Muscles need to work together like this so that joints don't get stuck in one position!

Walking may seem simple, but did you know that this action uses 200 muscles?

Ligaments hold bones together at the joint. They also stop joints being moved too far in one direction. You can use a protractor to measure the range of movement in various joints in your body, such as your arm, knee or thumb. You will find that some people have a much wider range of movement than others. Exercising muscles can increase their range. Ballet dancers, for example, train their bodies to become very flexible.

The human body contains more than 600 muscles. In adults, muscles make up nearly half the body weight.

If muscles are overworked, they can stay contracted for too long. This is called cramp.

14 Skin

Your skin is your largest organ, covering the whole of your body – even the inside of body openings such as your mouth and nose! Your skin is waterproof. It also protects your body from infections, injuries and the sun's harmful rays. The top layer of your skin consists of dead cells. Underneath, there are millions of tiny living cells. Each cell lives for about three weeks. As it grows older, it rises to the top of your skin and is rubbed off and replaced.

MAKE it WORK!
Make a model which will show you what goes on beneath your skin. Your skin not only protects your body, but also helps to control its temperature. Sweat **glands** pass sweat onto the surface of your skin. The sweat then **evaporates**, helping you to cool down.

You will need
dowels
a craft file
a felt-tip pen
blue, red and white wire
a polystyrene block
acrylic paint

1 Draw the rough shape of the skin cross-section on the block of polystyrene. Carefully carve out the shape using a craft file.

2 Shape the surface of the skin as shown. The hollows are the **pores**, which is where the sweat passes out.

3 Shape the layers of the skin as shown. You will see that there are three main layers. Carve the side of the cross-section, to make the three-dimensional shape of the sweat glands and hair **follicles**. The hairs on your body all grow out of follicles like these, buried under the top layers of your skin.

4 Push the dowels into the surface of the skin model. These represent the hairs which cover the entire surface of your body (except for the palms of your hands and soles of your feet).

5 Paint your model, using the different colours shown to represent the muscles, fatty tissue, sweat glands and hair follicles.

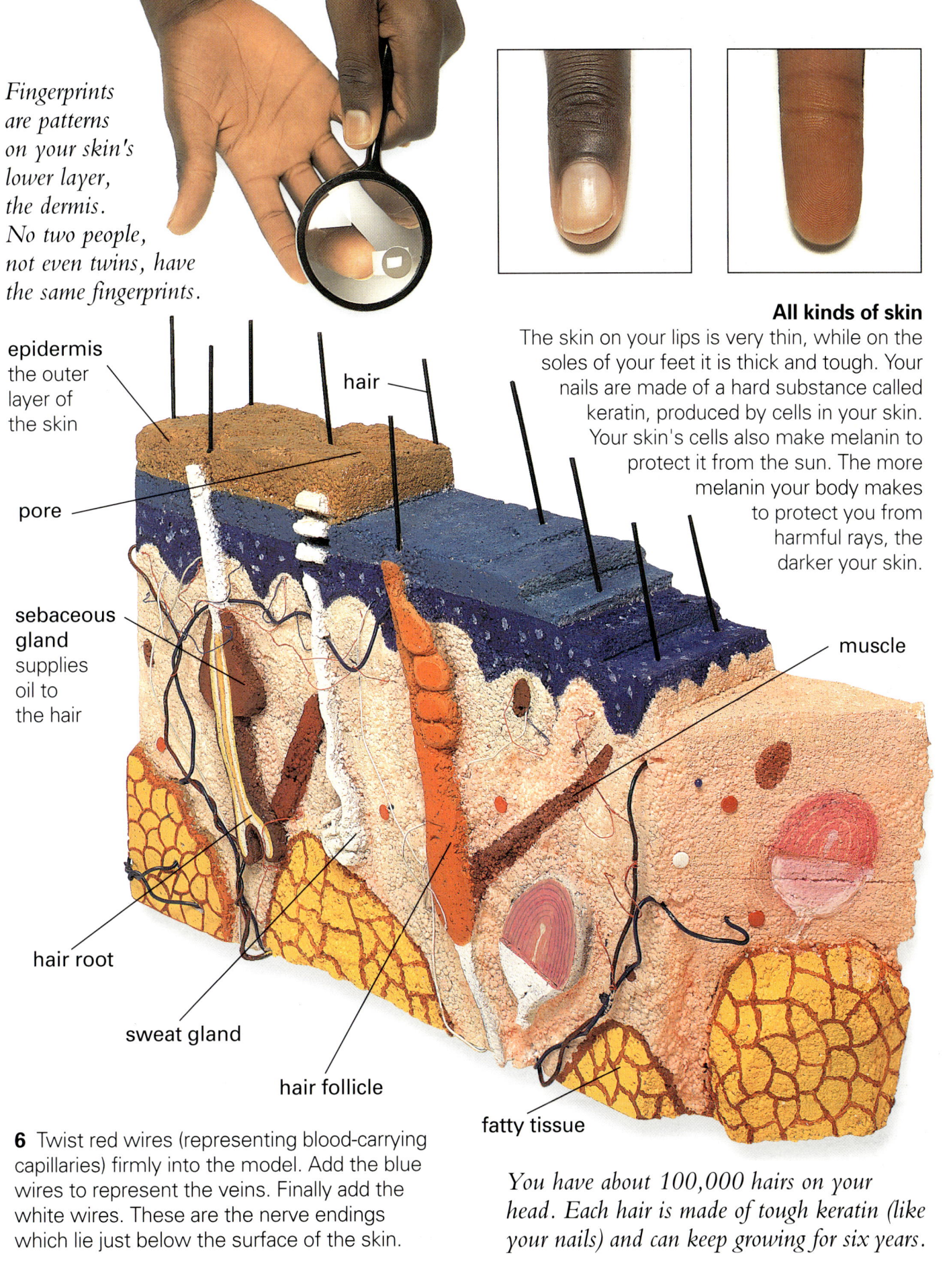

Fingerprints are patterns on your skin's lower layer, the dermis. No two people, not even twins, have the same fingerprints.

All kinds of skin
The skin on your lips is very thin, while on the soles of your feet it is thick and tough. Your nails are made of a hard substance called keratin, produced by cells in your skin. Your skin's cells also make melanin to protect it from the sun. The more melanin your body makes to protect you from harmful rays, the darker your skin.

epidermis the outer layer of the skin

pore

sebaceous gland supplies oil to the hair

hair

muscle

hair root

sweat gland

hair follicle

fatty tissue

6 Twist red wires (representing blood-carrying capillaries) firmly into the model. Add the blue wires to represent the veins. Finally add the white wires. These are the nerve endings which lie just below the surface of the skin.

You have about 100,000 hairs on your head. Each hair is made of tough keratin (like your nails) and can keep growing for six years.

16 Cells

Cells are the building blocks of the human body. Every part of your body – bones, skin, nerves, muscles – is made from cells. Although cells that do different jobs have different shapes and sizes, their basic structure is always the same.

Every single cell has its own control centre, or nucleus. This contains, in **chromosomes,** the instructions that the cell needs to keep on working.

▲ Humans belong to one big interelated group. They may not look related – they have different-coloured skin, hair and eyes. But they all belong to one species, or biological unit.

2 Cut a slot from the edge of each cardboard circle to its centre. Make the slot as wide as the thickness of the cardboard.

3 Slot the two cardboard circles together as shown and glue them into place. Paint them yellow.

4 Fold the circles in half, and glue them to the inside faces of your cardboard cell.

MAKE it WORK!
Make a model cross-section of a cell and see for yourself the complicated world it contains. It is hard to imagine that there are about 50,000 million cells in your body!

5 Use the foam ball to make the cell nucleus. Paint the outside of the ball green, then cut out a quarter-segment.

You will need
strong garden wire   electrical wire
thick cardboard   mapping pins
modelling clay   yellow paper
acrylic paint   a foam ball

6 Glue the ball to the wall of the cell as shown and paint the centre of the nucleus blue.

1 Cut two circles out of the cardboard. Then cut four matching circles out of the yellow paper.

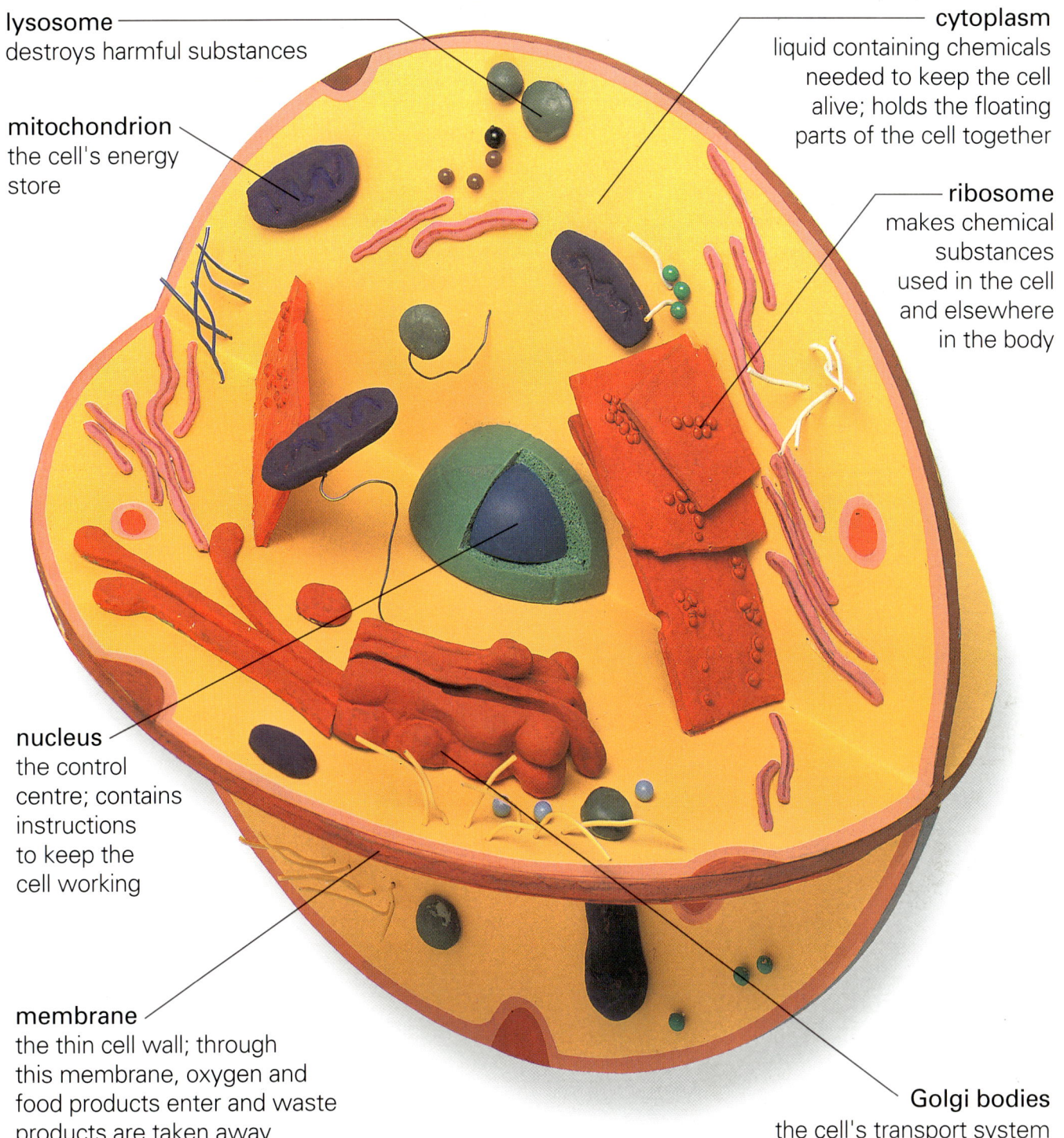

lysosome — destroys harmful substances

mitochondrion — the cell's energy store

cytoplasm — liquid containing chemicals needed to keep the cell alive; holds the floating parts of the cell together

ribosome — makes chemical substances used in the cell and elsewhere in the body

nucleus — the control centre; contains instructions to keep the cell working

membrane — the thin cell wall; through this membrane, oxygen and food products enter and waste products are taken away

Golgi bodies — the cell's transport system

7 With the modelling clay, shape all the other parts of the cell, using the photograph as a guide. Paint them. Push the pieces of electrical wire and mapping pins into the cardboard.

8 Use the strong garden wire to attach some of the floating parts of the cell to its walls. Glue the other parts straight onto the cardboard surface.

Most cells can reproduce themselves and will do so throughout your life. Some cells can only live for a few hours, days or weeks, but others last longer. Bone cells live for up to 20 years, while skin cells only live for three weeks. Your nerve cells cannot reproduce, so they have to last all your life.

18 The Nervous System

Millions of nerves make up your body's communication system. They carry electrical messages to and from your brain. Your brain and spinal cord operate the main organs of your body without you having to think about it. Your **sense** organs send messages to your brain about the outside world (see pages 36 to 41).

MAKE it WORK!
Make a model of the nervous system. You will see how nerves from all the main organs of the body are linked to the spinal cord. The spine sends messages directly between the body and the brain.

You will need
red and yellow paper
yellow cord
tape
glue

heart (p 22)
lung (p 24)

1 Take the spinal column which you have already made (see page 6).

2 Cut out 16 small discs and 3 larger oval shapes from yellow paper and 11 discs from red paper.

3 Cut 16 lengths of yellow cord.

▶ Fix yellow cord or wool to your clothes with small safety pins and make your own map of the central nervous system.

4 As you work through the book, make models of the body's organs and join them to the nervous system. Glue yellow cord to the red discs and attach the discs to the organs. Choose either male or female reproductive organs.

5 Thread the cord through the larger yellow discs, then knot it. These discs are like junctions, where nerves from several organs meet. Tape the nerves from the heart and lungs together.

6 Attach the remaining lengths of cord to the larger yellow discs as shown. Then stick the loose ends of the cords to the small yellow discs and glue these to the spine. The bones of the spine protect the delicate nerve endings.

stomach (p 28)
spleen (p 28)
small intestine (p 29)
penis and testicles (p 42)
kidney (p 30)
bladder (p 30)
gall bladder (p 28)
large intestine (p29)
liver (p 28)
spinal column (p 6)
uterus and vagina (p 42)

Sensory nerves
The nerves in your body constantly send messages about the outside world to your brain, which then sends back a response. For example, if you sip a cup of tea which is too hot, the nerves in your tongue send an urgent message to your brain. It then sends a message back along the nervous system to the muscles of your hand, telling them to put the cup down.

Your muscles sometimes work without your brain thinking about them. The movements they make are called **reflex** *actions and are controlled by the spinal cord alone, by-passing the brain. Try testing your reflexes. Sit in a chair with one leg crossed over the other. Ask a friend to tap your crossed leg just below the knee-cap. What happens to this leg?*

20 Blood

Your body contains five litres (almost nine pints) of blood which carries oxygen and digested food all over your body and collects waste. It is pumped around by your heart. Blood helps your body to fight infection and also to control how warm or cold you are by spreading heat as it travels around.

The blood transport system
The red and blue wool shows how blood is carried around the body in **blood vessels**. The arteries (shown in red) are the main highways of the blood system. They divide into smaller blood vessels. Tiny **capillaries** pass between the cells of the body, delivering oxygen from the lungs and food to every part.

Waste products are carried away in capillaries, which gradually join up to make veins (shown by the blue wool).

MAKE it WORK!
This model explains how blood is made up. It contains red cells, white cells, small fragments of cells called **platelets** and a liquid called **plasma**, in which the other blood cells float. Whenever we cut ourselves, platelets surround the wound and make a fine net, called fibrin, which seals the wound.

You will need
glue
a pan scrubber
a foam base block
five table-tennis balls
thin and thick sponge
lengths of thin wire
red and yellow paint

1 Paint the foam base black. Cut circles from the dishcloth to make platelets. Push a piece of wire into each platelet and then into the base.

2 Next, make the red blood cells. Cut out six doughnut-shaped pieces of sponge and paint them red. Attach them to the base with pieces of wire.

3 Now make the white blood cells. Paint the table-tennis balls and the pan scrubber yellow. Shred the pan scrubber. Tape a piece of wire to each ball, then cover it with some shredded scrubber. Push the wires into the base.

4 Take the rest of the shredded pan scrubber and spread it around the blood cells. This represents fibrin, which is made by the platelets.

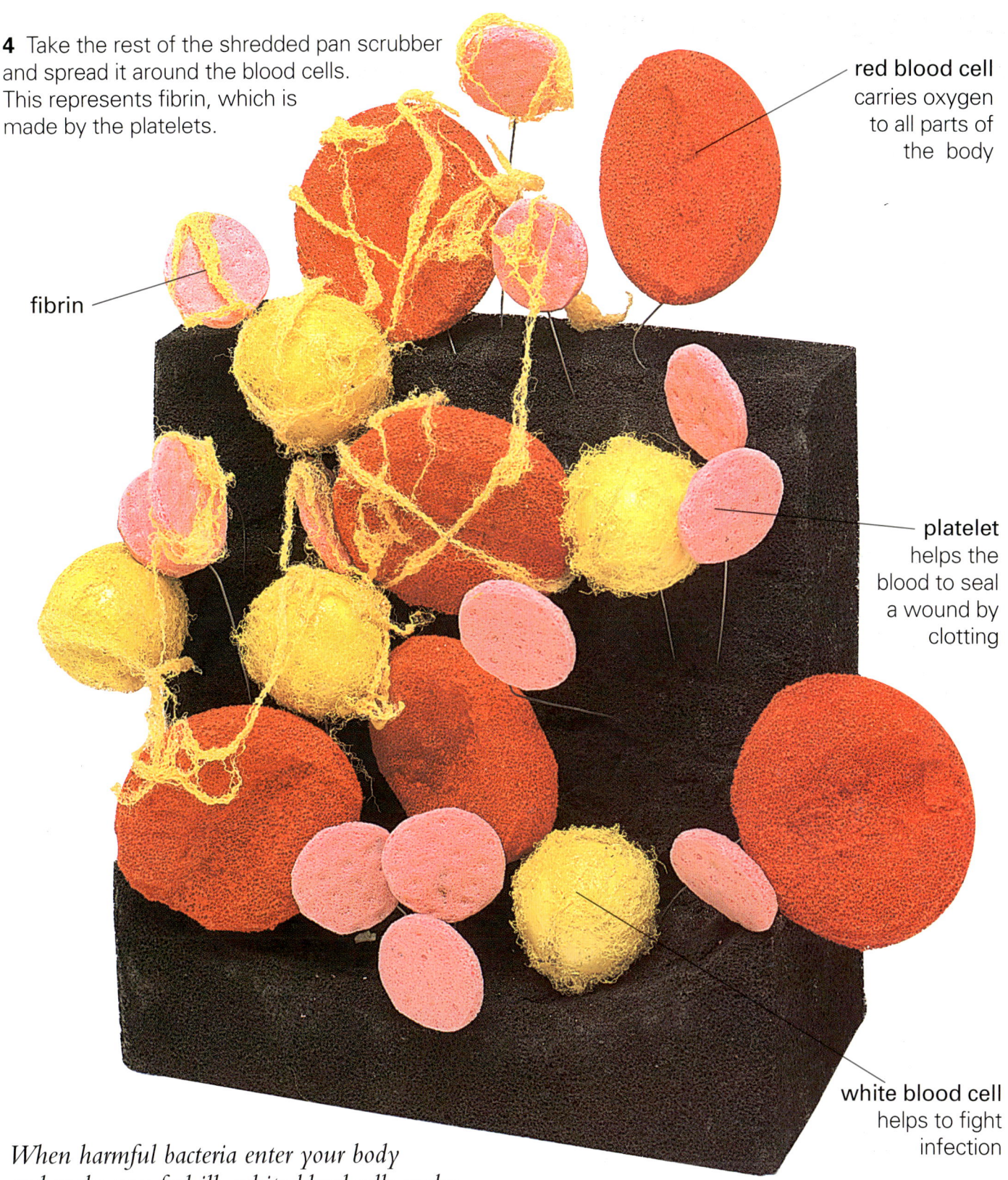

red blood cell carries oxygen to all parts of the body

fibrin

platelet helps the blood to seal a wound by clotting

white blood cell helps to fight infection

When harmful bacteria enter your body and make you feel ill, white blood cells make **antibodies**. *These attack the bacteria and stop them multiplying. When you are immunized, you are injected with a mild form of the poison produced by disease-causing bacteria.*

White blood cells react immediately by making antibodies. Your body is now ready to fight the real disease.

22 The Heart

Your heart is a muscle. Its job is to pump blood through blood vessels around your body. It has to repeat the same pumping action all your life, about once a second, to keep you alive. Blood containing oxygen is pumped through the left side of your heart to all parts of your body. When the oxygen has been used up, the blood is collected and sent back to the right side of your heart, and then to your lungs, ready to be filled with oxygen again.

▲ Cut out pieces of sponge and cardboard, glue them together and paint as shown. You will see that your model heart is divided into left and right sides, each with upper and lower chambers.

MAKE it WORK!
Make a pumping model to show how the four chambers in your heart work. Imagine how strong the muscle must be to repeat this action at least 60 times a minute!

You will need
four plastic bottles with screw-on tops
black tape
two bulldog clips
red and blue Plasticine
red and blue tape
two plastic funnels
red and blue food dye
two lengths of plastic tubing

1 Make small holes in the bottle tops. Cut two short lengths of plastic tube and push each end of both tubes into a bottle top. Seal the holes around the tubes with red and blue Plasticine.

2 Make holes in the base of two of the plastic bottles and in the sides of the other two.

3 Thread two longer pieces of plastic tubing through the holes in the side of the bottles. Make sure the tubes almost reach the bottom of the bottles. Seal the holes with Plasticine as before. Wrap red tape around the left-hand tube, and blue tape around the right-hand tube.

4 Now screw all four lids onto the bottles. Use black tape to fix the bottles together in pairs, making sure that those with holes in the base are upside down at the top.

5 Colour two jugs of water, one with blue and one with red food colouring. Blood which contains oxygen is red. Blue water represents blood returning to the heart for more oxygen.

6 Attach bulldog clips to the tubes which connect the two bottles. These will do the same job as the heart's **valves**. They are like swing-doors which only open one way. Once the blood has passed through the heart's upper chamber, the valves close.

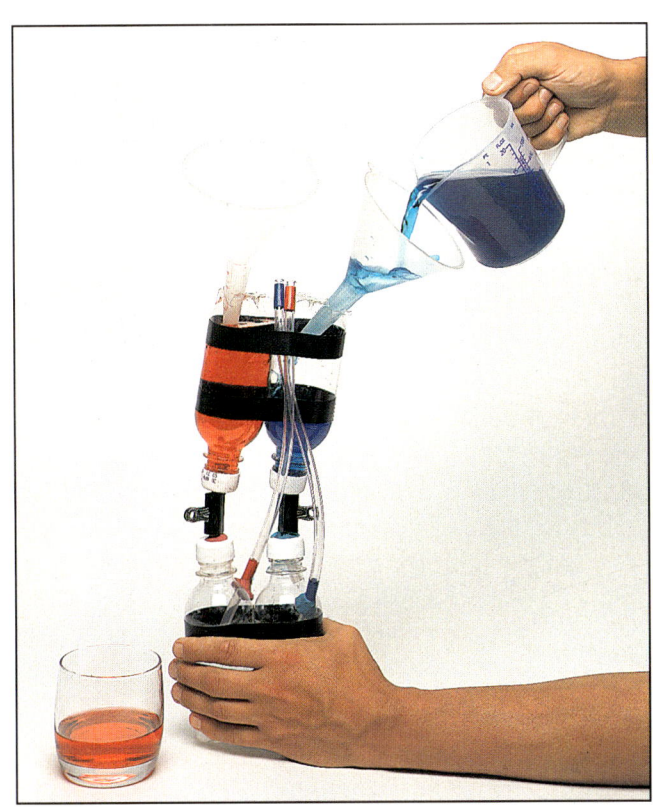

7 Using the funnels, carefully pour the red water into the bottle on the red side. Now pour blue water into the blue side. Open the bulldog clips to let the 'blood' run through the tubes, then close them.

8 Squeeze the lower bottles. This action is similar to the pumping of the heart. See how quickly the blood spurts out of the tubes, ready to be pumped all around the body.

Test your own or a friend's heartbeat. Find your pulse on the inside of your wrist, or at the side of your neck. When you feel it beating under your fingers, count how many beats you can feel in a minute. Take your pulse before and after doing some exercise. You will notice a big difference!

24 The Lungs

Your lungs have a very important job to do – they must absorb as much oxygen as possible from the air. We all need oxygen and also some carbon dioxide to keep us alive. Your body combines oxygen with the food you eat in order to release energy. When you breathe in, air is taken into your lungs. Oxygen is absorbed into the blood and is carried all over your body, through your blood vessels.

MAKE it WORK!
Did you know that adults' lungs hold about five litres (almost nine pints) of air? Find out your own lung capacity, or how much air your lungs can hold, by doing this simple experiment.

3 Place the palm of your hand over the open end of the bottle. Quickly turn it upside down and plunge it into the bowl. When you remove your hand, the water will stay in the bottle.

4 Tape the straws together. Slide one end under the bottle. Take a deep breath, and blow out into the other end of the straw.

5 Increased air pressure forces the water out of the bottle. Using your scale, measure the amount of air at the top of the bottle. This is your lung capacity. Now run on the spot for one minute, and try doing the experiment again. Does exercise affect your lung capacity?

You will need
a large bowl
a measuring jug
insulating tape
a plastic bottle
two straws

1 Fill the bowl with water. Cut the top off the plastic bottle. Fill the jug with water, and note down how many litres (pints) it contains.

2 Pour this water into the bottle. Using the tape, mark a scale (use 8-10 sections) up the side of the bottle.

A new-born baby's lungs are pink. As you get older, your lungs get blacker because of the polluted air they have to breathe. Lungs are very sensitive to the quality of air, so your body tries to protect them in all sorts of ways. Dry air is moistened by mucus in the nose as you breathe in. If the air is too cold, blood vessels in the nose will heat it up. Hairs in the nose trap particles of dust and dirt in the air before it reaches your lungs.

MAKE it WORK!

The lungs are not muscles. They expand when they are filled with air because of the action of the diaphragm, a flat muscle at the base of the ribs, and the chest wall. This experiment shows you how your diaphragm allows your lungs to breathe. The plastic bottle represents your chest, the straw is your throat, the yellow balloon is your diaphragm and the blue balloon is your lungs. As your diaphragm stretches and contracts, it inflates and deflates your lungs.

You will need

Plasticine
a blue balloon
two elastic bands
a small strip of wood
the upper half of a plastic bottle with lid
a yellow balloon
a straw

1 Cut the wood to fit the width of the bottle exactly. Glue it inside the cut end of the bottle.

2 Secure the yellow balloon over the open end of the bottle with an elastic band.

3 Make a small hole in the bottle top. Push the straw through. Fix the blue balloon onto the end of the straw with an elastic band. Seal the hole with Plasticine.

4 Screw the top back on the bottle with the blue balloon inside.

5 Stretch the yellow balloon downwards. This reduces the air pressure inside the bottle. More air is sucked in through the straw to fill the space, and inflates the blue balloon (your lungs).

6 Now push in the yellow balloon, to make the 'diaphragm' contract. The air pressure inside the bottle increases and forces air out through the straw. The blue balloon goes down. This is what happens when you breathe out.

▶ Make a pair of lungs by cutting out these foam shapes. Paint them as shown. The right-hand lung is a cross-section.

◀ Air passes down the branching tubes inside the lungs. It reaches air sacs, called **alveoli**. From here, the oxygen is passed into the blood.

26 Digestion

You begin **digesting** your food as soon as you put it in your mouth. This is just the start of its long journey. It will take about two days for the food to pass right through your digestive system. During this journey, your body will break the food down, until it has taken out the **nutrients** it needs.

You will need
a block of polystyrene
red, blue and green wires
red, blue and green straws
a felt-tip pen
acrylic paint
a craft file
sandpaper

1 Draw the molar on the polystyrene. Molars are large teeth at the back of the mouth, used for grinding food.

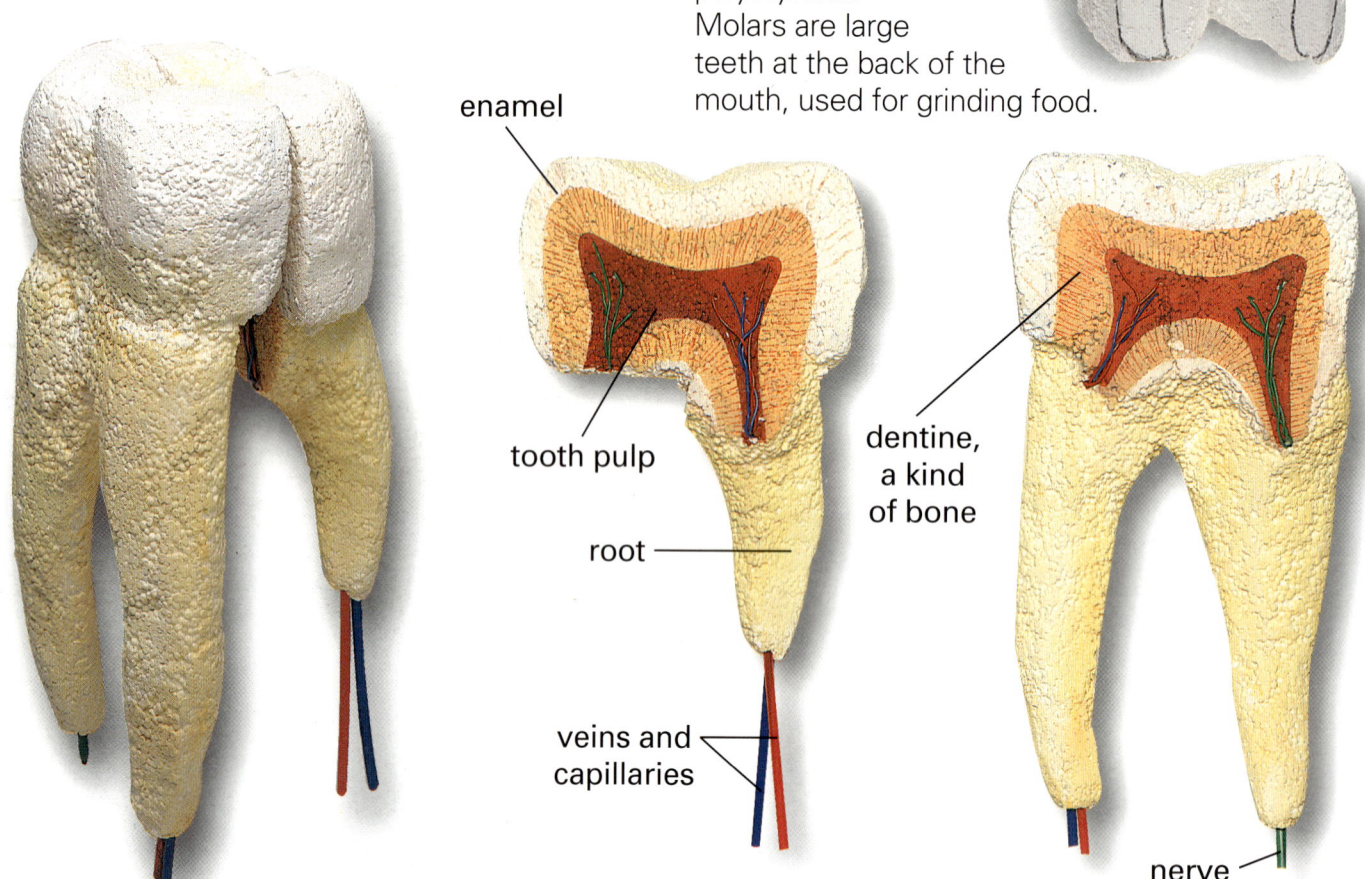

enamel

tooth pulp

root

veins and capillaries

dentine, a kind of bone

nerve

MAKE it WORK!
Your teeth are used in the first stage of your digestion. They chop, shred and grind up food in your mouth. Glands under your tongue make a liquid called **saliva**, which moistens the food and begins to break it down. When you have finished chewing your food, your tongue moves it to the back of your mouth. With one swallow your food starts its journey. Make a model molar and see what a tooth is like inside.

2 Carefully carve out the three roots. About a quarter of the way down the tooth, shape a ridge. Above this ridge, or gumline, the tooth is visible. Shape a ridge in the top of the tooth. Smooth down the polystyrene with sandpaper.

3 Now cut your molar in half to reveal the inside of the tooth. Paint it as shown. The enamel on the visible part of the tooth is whiter than the roots deep inside the gum.

4 Take the red and blue straws, which represent the capillaries and veins. Push them into the root of the tooth. Then take the blue and red wires and twist them around in the pulp cavity as shown. This is the soft centre of the tooth.

5 Do the same with the green straw and wire. This represents the tooth's nerve. If your tooth enamel decays, it can expose the nerve, which will give you toothache.

Human beings eat meat as well as vegetables, so we have teeth to suit both these kinds of food. At the front of our mouths, we have sharp, pointed teeth, which we use for tearing and shredding meat. Our large back teeth are used to grind vegetables. Animals such as cows only have grinding teeth because they eat only grass.

MAKE it WORK!
Make this model head to find out what the inside of your nose, mouth and throat look like. Use the labels to help you identify each part.

Sometimes your food 'goes down the wrong way.' This means that some food gets into your windpipe. When this happens, you start to choke. Air rushes up your windpipe very fast, pushing the food back into your mouth.

Bacteria live in your mouth because it is dark, warm and moist. They feed on sugars in your food and produce acids which can harm your teeth.

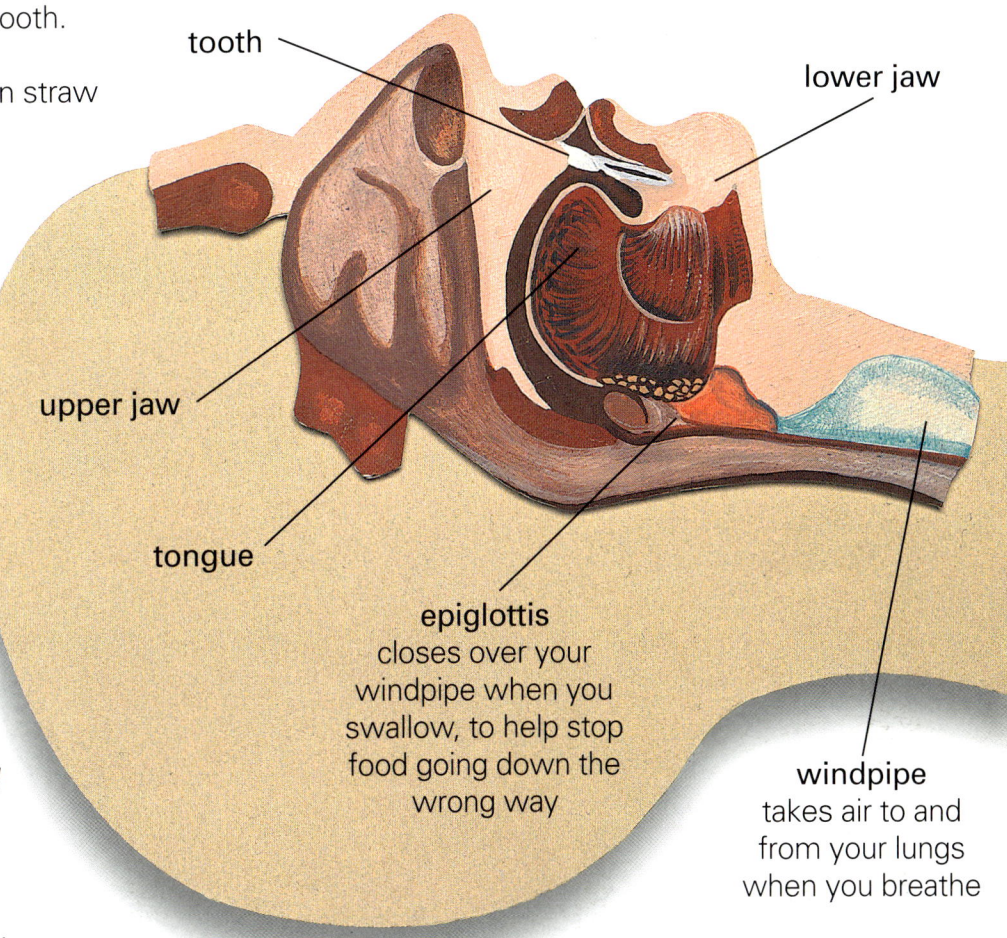

tooth
lower jaw
upper jaw
tongue
epiglottis closes over your windpipe when you swallow, to help stop food going down the wrong way
windpipe takes air to and from your lungs when you breathe

It is very important to brush your teeth as often as possible, as it is the only way to fight the germs which lurk between them and along your gums.

A good diet
Your food and drink provide your body with the things it needs to keep healthy. A balanced diet provides important vitamins and minerals. Proteins, found in meat, fish, eggs, milk, cheese and nuts, help you to grow. Carbohydrates, found in bread, sugar and potatoes, give you energy. Fibre, found in fruit and vegetables and whole grains, cannot easily be broken down. It helps to keep your digestive system working properly and passes out of your body as waste.

MAKE it WORK!
Make a life-size model digestive system. You will see that eating is just the start of all your body's hard work.

To support overlapping organs on your model, cut small squares of foam and paint them pink. Remember that the body does not have these!

1 Paint a cardboard base for your digestive system.

2 Cut out foam shapes for the liver, spleen and stomach, and paint them.

esophagus
the tube that leads from the mouth to the stomach pushes food down the tube by muscular movements

stomach
makes acid digestive juices which pour on food and begin to break down protein; food stays in the stomach for about two hours

liver
recieves nutrients from the blood, storing some and passing others on; also filters out poisons and uses energy from food to heat the blood

gall bladder (tucked underneath liver)
stores bile, which helps to break down fats and turn them into chemicals which can be absorbed through the intestine wall

spleen
helps fight infection, stores blood and removes worn-out red cells from blood

You will need
foam or sponge
pipe insulation
modelling clay
a felt-tip pen
acrylic paint
green wire
cardboard
Velcro

3 Make a cone out of modelling clay for the gall bladder, and paint it dark green. Push both green wires into the point of the cone and attach them at the other end to the liver.

4 Cut a grey cardboard base for the small intestine. Thread wire through a long strip of foam. Bend it into shape, paint it pink and glue it in place.

5 For the large intestine, cut the pipe insulation in half lengthwise, slice it up and glue the u-shaped pieces around the small intestine.

6 Stick the organs to the body base using Velcro discs.

large intestine
receives remains of food from the small intestine; waste products (including fibre, the part of food which is not digested) move down to the end of the intestine

rectum
the end of the large intestine; waste passes out through here when you go to the toilet to empty your bowels

small intestine
receives digested food from the stomach; chemicals from the food are absorbed into the bloodstream through the intestine wall

appendix
a dead end; not used by humans but helps certain animals to digest grass

If you eat too much food, or any food which is bad, your body has a very effective way of getting rid of it! The muscles of your stomach wall squeeze inwards and force the food back up your esophagus and out of your body. This is called vomiting or throwing up.

30 Purification

Water is vital to your body. Seventy per cent of your body weight is made up of water. Water carries important chemicals such as nutrients, as well as heat, around your body. You also absorb it when you eat, drink and breathe. You pass it out when you sweat and go to the toilet.

MAKE it WORK!
Make a model of your purification system. It includes your kidneys, two small bean-shaped organs found behind your waist. Tubes join them to your bladder, where urine is stored.

You will need
blue and red wire
sponge or foam
pipe cleaners
cardboard

kidney

ureter
tubes carrying urine from kidneys to bladder

nerves

blood vessels

bladder

Your kidneys work very efficiently to filter unwanted water and waste products from your blood. From these they make **urine**, a liquid which flushes waste out of the body. They process 150 litres (33 gallons) of water a day.

1 Cut foam shapes for the kidneys and bladder and a matching cardboard shape for the kidney in cross-section. Paint them as shown.

2 Cut out cardboard blood vessels and paint them blue and red. These blood vessels supply blood to the kidneys.

3 Attach the red and blue wires and pipe cleaners as shown. The wires are the nerves leading to and from your bladder. The pipe cleaners are the tubes which carry urine.

MAKE it WORK!

When blood passes through the kidneys, they act like a very fine sieve, filtering out waste products and purifying the blood. You can see how the kidneys work by doing this simple filtering experiment.

You will need

pieces of polystyrene
three strips of wood
food colouring
a plastic bottle
sand or soil
a glass tumbler
fine netting
a jug
tape

1 Ask an adult to help you slice three sections from the bottle.

2 Cut out ten circles of net – they should be slightly larger than the bottle sections.

3 Make three filters by taping the net to the bottle sections. Make one filter with just one piece of net, the second with three pieces of net, and the third with six pieces of net.

4 Glue the three strips of wood to the edge of the filters, as shown, so that they are free-standing.

5 Fill a jug with water. Then add food colouring (which contains very fine particles), sand or soil and chunks of polystyrene. These represent the different waste products in the blood when it arrives in the kidneys.

6 Pour the water through the filters and watch what happens. Everything except the finest food colouring particles is caught by the filters.

Sometimes, because of an accident or disease, the kidneys fail and cannot clean the blood. A special machine can be used to do their job. Blood is taken from an artery in the arm and passed through the machine, where it is cleaned and returned to the body. This is called dialysis. The blood has to pass through the machine 20 times before it is properly cleaned. Patients have to spend two 12-hour periods on the machine every week.

32 The Brain

Your brain is the control centre of your body. It runs all your body's functions and movements. It is also responsible for thoughts, memories and emotions.

Although it is quite small, your brain contains over 100,000 nerve cells. It uses up one fifth of your body's energy, so it needs a constant supply of oxygen.

1 Ask an adult to help you cut down the plastic ball so that it makes a neatly-fitting skullcap. This is the cortex, or outer layer of the brain.

2 Copy all the shapes shown on different coloured paper (see tip on page 8). These represent the different parts of the body that the brain controls.

MAKE it WORK!
Each part of the brain looks after different body functions. Make your own skullcap and plot which parts of your brain control which actions.

You will need
glue
pipe cleaners
half a plastic ball
coloured paper
paper fasteners

3 Bend the pipe cleaners in half and twist them. Glue a paper shape onto the bent end of each.

4 Make eight holes in the ball, following the photograph opposite. Push the open ends of each pipe cleaner through the right hole and bend the ends to fix it in position. Put on your skullcap to see exactly how your mind works!

movements — all your main muscular movements are controlled from here

touching — your brain receives signals from your skin here

hearing — messages from your ears are dealt with in this part of the brain

focus — this is where your brain makes pictures out of the messages received from your eyes

balance — this part of your brain makes sure you don't fall over!

eye muscles — this part of your brain controls the muscles around your eyes

speech — this part of your brain controls your voice box and the muscles of your mouth

hands — all your hand movements are controlled from here

The cortex of your brain is pinky-grey (it is known as 'grey matter'). It has the texture of firm jelly.

The brain stem is the part of your brain nearest to your spinal cord. It acts like an automatic pilot. It runs all your body's main systems, for example your digestion and circulation, and also your heart and lungs.

34 Memory

Everything you know about the world is stored in your brain. As you grow up, your brain processes everything that happens to you. Much of this is stored in your short-term memory and you will forget it quickly. For example, your memory of the pictures on the previous page will soon fade. Other experiences you remember for much longer because they are stored in your long-term memory. Everything you remember helps you to learn.

MAKE it WORK!
The brain helps us to understand what we see by remembering things we have seen before. But sometimes it can be fooled. This is known as an optical illusion. Make these illusions and confuse your friends!

You will need
thin black and coloured cardboard
a felt-tip pen
a ruler
scissors

▲ Using the ruler, cut two straight strips of dark coloured cardboard. Draw the pattern of straight lines on light cardboard and position the dark strips over it as shown. Do the dark lines look straight? The pattern of lines underneath has tricked your brain, making the dark strips look curved.

▲ Now cut out the two simple arrow shapes from light cardboard, as shown. Make sure that the centre lines are the same length. You will see that the arrowheads create an illusion. They make the centre lines look shorter and longer than they really are.

▲ Trace the outline of the left-hand side of the candlestick on coloured paper. Fold the paper in half and cut along the line. Unfold the paper and glue the candlestick to the centre of the black cardboard. As well as the candlestick, can you also see two faces looking at each other?

▶ Cut this shape from coloured cardboard. Is it a duck or a rabbit? Your brain can see only one image at a time.

MAKE it WORK!

This memory game is known as 'Kim's Game'. It's a good way to test your short-term memory. Try playing it with a friend and see how many objects each of you can remember. Can you find any way of helping your brain to memorize the objects more easily?

You will need
assorted everyday objects   pencil and paper
a tray or drawer
a cloth

2 Show the objects on the tray to a friend. Ask your friend to look at them for about a minute and try to memorize them, then cover the tray.

3 Give your friend a few moments to think, then see how many of the objects he or she can remember. Write them down and check them against the objects on the tray. Now try swapping places. Ask your friend to find a new set of objects and see how many of them you can remember.

1 Choose about 20 different small objects from around the house. Try to make sure that they are not connected with each other in any way (for example, do not choose objects which could all be found in your school desk). Lay everything out on the tray.

Ways to remember
The brain works better if you organize the things you are trying to remember. You could do this by putting them in alphabetical order, arranging them by colour, or even making up a story about them. Maybe you will find that your brain works better in pictures. You can take a number of different objects and make a crazy picture out of them in your mind's eye. Try playing 'Kim's Game' using these ways of remembering and see whether you can improve your score.

Most people can only remember a maximum of nine numbers. That is why telephone numbers have only up to seven digits. If they were longer, no-one would remember them!

36 Sight

There are five main senses – sight, hearing, touch, smell and taste. They send vital information to your brain about the world around you. Your eyes are the sense organs that receive information in the form of light rays bouncing off everything you look at. Your eyes turn these rays into messages that your brain can understand.

You will need

red and blue wire
a magnifying glass
an old plastic football
thick and thin dowels
a clear plastic bottle
sticky tape
a flashlight
acrylic paint
thin cardboard
corrugated cardboard

1 Ask an adult to help you cut the football in half, trim the flat base from the plastic bottle and cut short pieces of thick and thin dowel in half lengthways with a sharp knife or saw.

The eye is shaped like a ball and contains a jelly-like fluid. It has a clear covering (the cornea) at the front. The coloured part of the eye is called the iris and has a small hole at its centre (the pupil), through which light enters. The lens is behind the pupil and it focuses light on the retina, a special lining at the back of the eyeball. The retina detects the light rays and turns them into messages which it sends to the brain along the optic nerve.

MAKE it WORK!
Make this model eye and see for yourself how your eyes are your windows on the world!

2 Paint the inside of one half of the ball red, with lighter red and blue veins. This represents the retina.

3 Cut out the cardboard shapes and paint them as shown. Glue them together, placing the red muscles at the top and bottom. Tape the cardboard shape around the edge of the football half.

4 Twist the blue and red wires together and stick one end inside the football, as shown. Glue the dowels together, paint them, then stick them in position on the cardboard. This is the optic nerve, joining the eye to the brain.

5 Slot the magnifying glass and bottle base into position in the cardboard surround, as shown. They represent the lens and the cornea.

Your pupils control the amount of light entering your eyes. Look at yourself in a mirror in a dimly-lit room. Your pupils, the black spots in the middle of your eyes, will be quite large. This helps them to let in as much light as possible so that you can see the room. Now turn on the light and notice how quickly your pupils react to the light, by getting smaller.

JOHN MARSHALL SCHOOL
3910 ST. JAMES AVE.
NIAGARA FALLS, ONTARIO

retina

cornea

pupil

lens

optic nerve

6 Shine the flashlight through the cornea. You can see how the lens focuses light on the retina.

The shape of the lens is altered by muscles, so that it can focus images clearly. When you look at a distant image, your lens is long and thin. To focus on a close image, it becomes short and fat. Sometimes the lens muscles do not work properly and images look blurred and fuzzy. This problem is helped by wearing more lenses, such as glasses or contact lenses, to correct the focus.

38 Taste and Smell

Your sense of smell helps you to recognize things at a distance, while your sense of taste detects the flavours of food and drink. You use both senses to check that food is fresh and will not harm you. Taste buds on your tongue's surface detect how salty, sweet, sour or bitter food is when it is mixed with saliva. Tiny hairs inside your nose pick up scent particles in the air and tell you about the flavour of food, too. If you have a blocked nose, you usually lose most of your sense of taste.

▼ Blindfold your friend. First, put a few drops of each liquid on their tongue, and see if they can recognize whether it is bitter, sweet, sour or salty. Write down the answers.

Certain parts of your tongue are more sensitive to some foods than others, because different taste buds detect different flavours. In general, the sweet and salty taste buds are near the front of the tongue. Sour and bitter taste buds are at the back and sides.

Experiment with putting the liquids on different parts of your friend's tongue. Note down their guesses and see if this is true.

MAKE it WORK!
How good is your sense of taste? Wine-tasters can tell the difference between many different flavours. Can you recognize the four main flavours – bitter, sweet, sour and salty – when you are blindfolded?

You will need
a blindfold   a teaspoon
water for rinsing the teaspoon between tests
samples of sweet, salty, sour and bitter liquids, for example sugar in water, salt in water, lemon juice in water and black coffee

Our food and drink has many variations on sweet, salty, sour and bitter tastes. We pick these up from the smell of the things we eat and without the sense of smell, it can be difficult to tell foods apart. Experiment with this by asking your friend to hold their nose. Give them a piece of apple and a piece of onion to eat. Can they tell what they're eating?

Your tongue isn't just used for tasting. It moves food around so your teeth can chew it and pushes the food to the back of your mouth, ready for swallowing.

MAKE it WORK!

Make a gigantic model tongue in polystyrene, and find out exactly where the different types of taste buds are found.

1 Using the craft file, cut out the polystyrene in the shape shown. Paint the tongue pink.

2 Cut out the bubble wrap in the shape of the tongue and paint it pink. Position it on the tongue model.

You will need
thumbtacks in four different colours
a sheet of bubble wrap
acrylic paint
polystyrene
a craft file
glue

sweet taste buds

bitter taste buds

sour taste buds

salty taste buds

Scent particles are chemicals which float around in the air we breathe. Humans can recognize about 3,000 separate smelly chemicals and many more smells that are combinations of these.

3 Stick the different-coloured thumbtacks through the bubble wrap and into the tongue, as shown. These show where the sweet, salty, sour and bitter taste buds are located.

40 Touch and Hearing

Nerve endings all over your skin give you a sense of touch. They notice heat and cold, texture, pressure and pain. Your sense of hearing can alert you to things you may not have seen, or that are out of reach. It also helps you to communicate with other people.

1 Put the first finger of your left hand into the hot water, and the first finger of your right hand into the cold water.

2 Wait for about a minute then, one at a time, dip each finger into the warm water.

3 The finger from the hot water feels cold, because it senses a drop in temperature. The finger from the cold water will feel warm, because it senses a temperature increase.

MAKE it WORK!
Test how your skin reacts to heat and cold and changes in temperature by doing this simple experiment. Not all parts of your skin have the same number of nerves. Fingertips, toes and lips are the most sensitive parts of the body.

You will need
a glass of warm water   a glass of cold water
a glass of hot tap water

Blind people are able to read using a system called braille. Patterns of raised bumps, representing letters and words, are made on the page. The blind person can read what is written by touching the bumps with their fingertips, which are especially sensitive. This system of writing was invented in 1824 by a Frenchman, Louis Braille, who became blind at the age of three.

MAKE it WORK!
Try the blindfold test, and see how much you can find out using only your sense of touch.

You will need
a large cardboard box
assorted objects
a large cloth

1 Turn the box on its side, and make a hole in the base large enough to put your hands through. Drape the cloth over the box.

2 Place various objects in the box. Try to choose things which have a different feel. For example, a spoon is hard and metallic, wool is soft, a brush is bristly.

3 Try the touch test on a friend. When they put their hands through the slot, they will not be able to see the objects. Ask them to describe what they are touching.

Hearing
Sounds are made by air vibrating. Your ears act as sound collectors, picking up these vibrations and trapping them in your outer ear. From here, the sounds pass down to your ear-drum, which is a very thin piece of skin separating your outer ear from your middle ear. The ear-drum vibrates in turn, passing the sound on to three small bones in your middle ear. One of these, the tiny stirrup bone, is about the size of a grain of rice! The vibrations are then passed into the fluid inside your inner ear, deep inside your skull. From here they are converted into electrical signals and passed on to your brain.

Is it soft? Is it rough? Is it cold and hard like metal? What shape is it? Can they guess what the object is? Now ask your friend to place some different objects in the box. How many of these can you identify?

The brain is able to separate sounds into those you want to hear and background noises. You can often hear your friend talking even though a huge truck is thundering past.

42 Reproduction

The nucleus of every cell in your body contains a set of coded instructions, called genes. These are made from a special chemical called DNA. Genes affect how you look, your character and your abilities. You inherit genes from your parents.

MAKE it WORK!

When two sets of genes combine to make a new life, a sperm cell made in the father's testes has to fertilize an egg cell from the mother's ovaries. The baby grows for 38 weeks inside a stretchy, muscular sac called the uterus.

1 To make models of the male and female reproductive organs, cut the shape of the body bases from light cardboard and paint them as shown.

bladder

vagina   uterus

testicle   penis

When a sperm from a male fertilizes an egg from a female, a new life begins. A set of genes from the mother and one from the father are brought together in one cell. This cell now contains all the instructions needed to make a new human being, although it is no bigger than a pinhead. As the baby develops, and new cells grow, the pattern from the parents' genes is repeated again and again. We call this heredity. It is not surprising that family members often look alike!

2 Cut the shapes of the reproductive organs out of foam. Paint them like the ones in the photograph and attach them to the male and female bases with Velcro.

You will be amazed by what we inherit from our parents. Apart from obvious things like the shape of your face and features and your height, some very odd things are passed on in the genes. 'Double-jointed' thumbs, which bend back to the wrist, are hereditary. So is the ability to roll your tongue up at the edges. How many of your friends have these genes?

MAKE it WORK!

How many characteristics do you share with the rest of your family? You are not exactly like them. With every generation, new sets of genes are introduced into a family. Play the generation game and see for yourself the vast number of variations that are possible.

You are a combination of your mother's and father's genes. If their genes are different, for example for eye colour, one colour may be dominant, or stronger than the other. If you inherit genes for both brown and blue eyes, you will have brown eyes, as the brown-eye gene is dominant.

1 Using Plasticine or modelling clay (which you can then paint), make two shapes, such as a ball and a cube. These will represent the first generation of your family.

2 What happens as these shapes combine to make new shapes in the next generation?

Scientists only began to discover how genetic codes worked in the 1950s. All over the world today, scientists are working to understand the way genes make up the human body.

3 Introduce a different shape to the second generation. How will it affect the third generation? One generation may produce a set of identical twins. The fertilized egg has divided to make two babies who share exactly the same genes.

Genes can contain instructions that make your body go wrong. Many serious illnesses are hereditary. Hemophilia stops the blood from clotting and is passed on by mothers, who rarely suffer from the disease, to their sons.

44 The Whole Body

Your body is an efficient, smooth-running machine. By now, you will have seen that it contains a number of different systems, each with its own job to do. These systems keep your body running from day to day. Food and oxygen are taken in, carried in your blood and used as a source of energy. Your body gets rid of waste products efficiently. Messages are carried back and forth between your brain and the outside world. But your body also has to deal with problems. It is the job of your defence or **immune** system to fight infection and mend or repair your body when things go wrong.

▶ Now that you have made all your main body systems, you can lay them out and see how they work together.

Skin
The skin helps to control the body's temperature. It protects the organs of the body, and is also the organ of touch.

Skeleton
The 206 bones of the body provide a framework and protect important organs. Red blood cells are made in the bone marrow.

Muscles
The muscles are responsible for moving the body. Involuntary muscles also keep other body systems (such as the digestion) running smoothly.

Nervous system
This system consists of the brain, spinal cord, nerves and sense organs. Nerves carry messages to and from the brain. The nervous system controls all the body's activities.

Blood
The blood system consists of the heart, blood and blood vessels. Blood transports oxygen and nutrients to the cells, and takes away waste products. White blood cells also protect you from disease.

Breathing
The lungs are responsible for taking in the oxygen from the air you breathe, and passing it into your blood.

Digestion
This system is one long tube through which food passes. It starts at your mouth and ends at your rectum. Organs such as the liver, gall bladder and pancreas help to break the food down and extract nutrients from it.

Purification
Your kidneys purify the blood and get rid of waste.

Things that go wrong

When you think how much your body has to do, it seems amazing that it runs so smoothly. When things do go wrong, your body will try its best to put them right.

Bacteria are tiny living organisms. They live all around us, and are often harmless. Some bacteria, however, reproduce very rapidly inside your body and can make you feel ill, as they produce poisons. Infected wounds, food poisoning and tonsillitis are all examples of illnesses caused by bacteria.

Broken bones: a bad fall or accident can sometimes break or fracture bones in your body. A broken bone can be 'set' by being held back in its correct position in a plaster cast. The bone on either side of the break then knits together, repairing the damage. An accident may also pull a joint out of place, or **dislocate** it. A doctor can move the bones back into the correct position.

Although many things can go wrong with a complicated machine like the human body, modern medicine can put many things right. Over the centuries medicine has made great progress. The 20th century in particular has seen many important advances and people now live longer than in the past. Scientists are still working to find cures for diseases such as AIDS and cancer, and exciting new discoveries about the body are still being made.

Viruses are tiny **organisms** which invade the body's cells. Once they are inside a cell, they change it into a mini-factory which produces more and more viruses. Eventually the cell bursts and dies, releasing the new viruses into the body.

Viruses cause a huge range of diseases – from the common cold to influenza, chicken pox and measles. The body fights viruses by producing antibodies in the white blood cells – often this process can make you feel ill, too.

As a human body grows older, its systems begin to slow down. Cells renew themselves more slowly, the skin wrinkles and muscles become looser. The senses are less sharp and the body finds it harder to fight disease. But these signs of ageing go hand in hand with gaining a lifetime of knowledge and experience, which can help us enjoy old age.

46 Glossary

Alveoli Tiny sacs in your lungs where oxygen is collected and absorbed into the blood.

Antibodies Substances in your blood which destroy the harmful bacteria and viruses that cause diseases.

Blood vessel Any of the different tubes, such as veins and arteries, through which blood circulates around your body.

Capillary A tiny blood vessel which links larger ones and carries blood to and from your cells.

Cell Cells are the basic building blocks which make up your body. Each cell has a centre, or nucleus, which contains the instructions it needs to do its job.

Chemical Chemicals are substances from which all things are made. There are many different chemicals in the human body.

Chromosome The nucleus of every cell contains structures called chromosomes, which carry genes. The genes control all the characteristics we inherit from our parents.

Digesting The action of breaking down food into chemicals which your body can absorb and can send to your cells to produce energy.

Dislocate A joint is dislocated when a bone is pushed out of place so the joint does not work.

Evaporate When a liquid changes into a gas, it evaporates.

Follicle A small pocket in your skin. Every hair on your body grows out of its own follicle.

Gland A cell or organ which either makes chemicals for your body to use or helps to remove waste products from your body. For example sweat glands remove water, passing sweat out onto the surface of your skin.

Immune Your immune system helps your body to fight disease and infection. When you have successfully fought off certain diseases, such as mumps, you become immune. Your body will be able to resist the disease if it attacks again.

Involuntary Many parts of your body work without you having to think about them. Involuntary muscles keep body systems such as breathing and circulation running smoothly.

Joint The point where two bones meet. There are many different types of joints which allow your body to move in a variety of ways.

Keratin A hard substance made in the cells of your hair, skin and nails.

Ligament A tough, elastic band of tissue which holds bones together at a joint.

Marrow A soft, jelly-like substance found inside most bones, where red blood cells and some white blood cells are made.

Melanin A coloured substance in your skin which darkens it and protects it against the Sun's harmful rays.

Metacarpal A bone which connects your finger or thumb to your wrist.

Muscle Muscles are made from strong, elastic tissue. They move the parts of your body.

Nutrient A chemical which your body extracts from food to give it energy to grow and work.

Organ A group of tissues which form a shape and work together to do a particular job in the body, for example the heart or liver.

Organism An organism is a living being.

Platelet A minute particle in the blood. When you cut your skin, platelets surround the wound and make a fine net, or clot, which stops you from bleeding.

Plasma The liquid part of your blood in which red and white blood cells and platelets float.

Pore A tiny opening in the surface of the skin through which substances such as sweat pass.

Reflex An automatic response in your body, such as blinking or a knee-jerk. You cannot stop a reflex by thinking about it.

Saliva A liquid produced by glands in your mouth. It moistens food, making it easier to swallow, and begins the chemical process of digestion, by helping to break food down.

Sense The main senses are sight, smell, hearing, taste and touch. They help you to find out about the world around you. Your brain receives messages from your sense organs: your eyes, nose, ears, tongue and skin.

Skeletal Attached to the skeleton. Skeletal muscles move your bones and are responsible for body movements that you have to think about, such as walking.

Skeleton The bony framework which supports your body and protects delicate organs such as your heart and brain.

Species A group of plants or animals whose members share the same characteristics and can breed together successfully.

Tendon Special tissue which attaches your muscles to your bones.

Tissue A collection of cells, usually of the same type, which work together to make up a part of the body. For example, the skin is a type of tissue made up of many cells.

Urine A liquid made up of waste water and chemicals from the blood. It is made in the kidneys, passed down to the bladder and then leaves your body via a tube called the urethra.

Valve Your veins and heart contain valves to stop blood from flowing backwards. They open in one direction only. When blood has passed through them, they flap shut like swing doors.

48 Index

antibodies 21
appendix 29
arteries 20

backbone – *see* spine
bacteria 21, 27, 45
balance 6, 33
bladder 7, 30, 42
blood 20–21, 22, 24, 25, 28, 29, 30, 31, 43, 44
bones 4, 6–7, 8, 9, 10, 11, 12, 13, 16, 19, 41, 44, 45
Braille, Louis 40
brain 7, 8, 10, 18, 19, 32–33, 34, 35, 36, 41, 44
breathing 24, 25, 30, 44

capillaries 20, 26
cartilage 9, 10
cells 4, 7, 14, 15, 16–17, 20, 21, 28, 32, 42, 44, 45
chromosomes 16
cortex 32, 33

diaphragm 25
diet 27
digestive system 12, 26–29, 33, 44
DNA 42

ears 8, 9, 33, 41, 43
epiglottis 27
esophagus 28, 29
eyes 8, 9, 33, 36–37

fingernails 15
fingerprints 15

gall bladder 28, 44
genes 42, 43

hemophilia 43
hairs 14, 24, 38
hearing 41
heart 4, 5, 7, 20, 22–23, 33, 44
heredity 42, 43
hips – see pelvis

infection 14, 20, 28, 44
intestines 28, 29

joints 6, 9, 10–11, 13, 45

kidneys 30–31, 44

ligaments 6, 10, 13
lips 15, 40
liver 28, 44
lungs 5, 7, 20, 22, 34–35, 27, 33, 44

mammals, characteristics of 4, 6, 7
membrane 17, 41
memory 32, 34–35
movement 5, 6, 10, 11, 13, 32, 33
mucus 24
muscles 4, 6, 12–13, 16, 19, 22, 25, 29, 33, 37, 44

nerves 16, 17, 18, 40, 44
nervous system 18–19, 40, 44
nose 9, 14, 24, 38
nutrients 26, 28, 30, 44

ovaries 42
oxygen 17, 20, 21, 22, 24, 25, 32, 44

pancreas 44
pelvis 6, 7, 11
rectum 29, 44
reflexes 19
reproduction 42–43
ribs 7, 25

saliva 26, 38
senses 18, 19, 33, 36–41, 44, 45
skin 5, 6, 14–15, 16, 33, 40, 44, 45
skull 7, 8–9, 10, 41
smell 38–39
sperm 42
spinal cord 18, 19, 33, 44
spine 6, 10, 18, 19,
spleen 28
stomach 28, 29
sweating 14, 15, 30

taste 38–39
teeth 8, 9, 26, 27, 38
tendons 12,
testes 42
thumb 7, 11, 42
toes 6, 40
tongue 19, 26, 27, 38, 39, 42
touch 40
twins 43

uterus 42

veins 20
virus 45

windpipe 27